ICS 67.140.10

SCM

世界中医药学会联合会
World Federation of Chinese Medicine Societies

SCM 0027-2019

凉茶饮料

Liang Cha (Herbal Beverage)

世界中联国际组织标准 2019-05-13发布实施
International Standard of WFCMS Issued & implemented on May 13th, 2019

中医古籍出版社
Publishing House of Ancient Chinese Medical Books

图书在版编目（CIP）数据

凉茶饮料：汉英对照 / 世界中医药学会联合会著
.—北京：中医古籍出版社有限公司，2019.11（2020.1 重印）
ISBN 978-7-5152-1951-6

Ⅰ.①凉… Ⅱ.①世… Ⅲ.①茶剂—中草药—配方—标准—汉、英 Ⅳ.① R283.6-65

中国版本图书馆 CIP 数据核字（2019）第 229006 号

凉茶饮料

世界中医药学会联合会　著

责任编辑　王晓曼
出版发行　中医古籍出版社有限公司
社　　址　北京东直门内南小街 16 号（100700）
电　　话　010-64089446（总编室）010-64002949（发行部）
网　　址　www.zhongyiguji.com.cn
印　　刷　北京建宏印刷有限公司
开　　本　880mm×1230mm　1/16
印　　张　1.25
字　　数　49 千字
版　　次　2019 年 11 月第 1 版　2020 年 1 月第 2 次印刷
书　　号　ISBN 978-7-5152-1951-6
定　　价　36.00 元

目　次

前　言

本标准的主要起草单位：通标标准技术服务有限公司广州分公司

本标准参与起草的单位：广州王老吉药业股份有限公司、广州王老吉大健康产业有限公司、北京同仁堂（亳州）饮片有限责任公司、深圳市深晖企业有限公司、中山市百怡饮料有限公司、普宁益君嘉食品有限公司、广西至臻投资有限公司、南阳市誉兴饮料有限公司、TRISTAR FOOD WHOLESALE CO INC.（美国）、SHENG SHENG F&B INDUSTRIES PTE LTD.（新加坡）

本标准主要起草人：李楚源、郑荣波、徐文流、方广宏、杨潞芳、黄晓丹、冯小清、丘燕、翁少全、伍柏坚、彭绍忠、李词周、朱焕容、沈颖莉、张丰源、Ivan Chan（中国香港）、任志正（中国台湾）、Michael G. Lien（美国）、Charles Chua（新加坡）

本标准参与起草人及审阅专家：

中　　国：李振吉、林瑞超、陈震、韩晶岩、付强、何洁仪、魏金明、刘馨磊、陈文锐、苏彩珠、罗佳妮

加 拿 大：程昭

西 班 牙：陈月龄、Ramon M. Calduch

澳大利亚：刘炽京

匈 牙 利：Gábor Nagy、于福年、夏林军

乌 克 兰：Samsonov

伊　　朗：Amir Hooman Kazemi

加　　蓬：Ovonon Komo

巴　　西：Reginaldo de Carvlaho Silva

以 色 列：Tuvia Scott

意 大 利：陈辉

新 西 兰：崔鹏德

美　　国：Deborah Lincoln、田海河

本标准的起草程序遵守了世界中医药学会联合会发布的 SCM 0001–2009《标准制定和发布工作规范》。

前 言

凉茶饮料

1 范围

本标准适用于 3.1 定义的预包装凉茶饮料。

2 规范性引用文件

下列文件对本标准的应用是必不可少的。凡是注日期的引用文件，仅注日期的版本适用于本标准。凡是不注日期的引用文件，其最新版本（包括所有的修改版）适用于本标准。

GB 4789.26《食品安全国家标准 · 食品微生物学检验 · 商业无菌检验》

GB 5009.268《食品安全国家标准 · 食品中多元素的测定》

GB 5009.22《食品安全国家标准 · 食品中黄曲霉毒素 B 族和 G 族的测定》

GB 5009.96《食品安全国家标准 · 食品中赭曲霉毒素 A 的测定》

GB/T 22388《原料乳与乳制品中三聚氰胺检测方法》

CAC/GL66 *Guidelines for the use of flavourings*

CODEX STAN 192 *General standard for food additives*

CODEX STAN 193 *General standard for contaminants and toxins in food and feed*

AOAC 932.14 *Solids in syrups by means of refractometer*

AOAC 990.28 *Sulfites in foods optimized Monier-Williams method*

ISO 4833–1 *Microbiology of the food chain—Horizontal method for the enumeration of microorganisms —part 1: Colony count at 30℃ by the pour plate technique*

ISO 4832 *Microbiology of food and animal feeding stuffs —Horizontal method for the enumeration of coliforms—Colony-count technique*

ISO 6579–1 *Microbiology of the food chain —Horizontal method for the detection, enumeration and serotyping of Salmonella —part 1: Detection of Salmonella spp.*

FDA/BAM chapter 4 *Enumeration of Escherichia coli and the Coliform Bacteria*

AOAC 975.55 *Staphylococcus aureus in foods-surface plating method for isolation and enumeration*

ISO 18662–1 *Traditional Chinese medicine —Vocabulary —Part 1: Chinese Materia Medica*

ISO 18664 *Traditional Chinese Medicine —Determination of heavy metals in herbal medicines used in Traditional Chinese Medicine*

ISO 21371 *Traditional Chinese medicine —Labelling requirements of products intended for oral or topical use*

FDA/BAM chapter 18 *Yeasts, Molds and Mycotoxins*

3 术语和定义

下列术语和定义适用于本标准。

3.1 凉茶饮料

基于传统中医药养生理论，以仙草、鸡蛋花、布渣叶、菊花等的一种或多种为原料，添加或不添加其他植物原料或提取物、其他辅料或食品添加剂，经提取、浓缩、配制、灭菌、灌装（或灌装、灭菌）、包装等主要工艺加工制成的预包装饮料。

4 技术要求

4.1 原辅材料要求

应符合相关国家或地区对使用原辅材料标准及法规要求。

4.2 感官要求

产品应具有标签标示的植物原料制成饮料所特有的色泽、气味、滋味等。

4.3 理化要求

应符合表 1 的规定

表 1 理化要求

项目	限值要求
可溶性固形物	≥0.5g/L
二氧化硫残留量	≤10mg/L

4.4 食品添加剂

应符合相关国家或地区对饮料类型产品的食品添加剂使用要求。

4.5 污染物要求

应符合表 2 的规定。

表 2 污染物要求

类别	项目	限制要求
重金属	砷	≤0.1mg/L
	铅	≤0.2mg/L
	汞	≤0.05mg/L
	铜	≤2.0mg/L
	锡（仅适用于金属罐装产品）	≤150mg/L
真菌毒素	赭曲霉毒素 A	≤5μg/L
	总黄曲霉毒素（B1、B2、G1、G2 之和）	≤5μg/L

4.6 微生物指标

4.6.1 以罐头加工工艺生产的产品应符合商业无菌的要求。

4.6.2 其他包装的产品微生物指标应符合表 3 的规定。

表 3　微生物要求

项目	采样方案及限量要求			
	n	c	m	M
菌落总数 (CFU/mL)	5	0	200	/
大肠菌群 (CFU/mL)	5	0	0	/
霉 菌 (CFU/mL)	≤ 20			
酵母菌 (CFU/mL)	≤ 20			
沙门氏菌 (CFU/25mL)	5	0	0	/
金黄色葡萄球菌 (CFU/mL)	5	1	100	1000
大肠杆菌 (CFU/mL)	5	0	0	/

注：

n: 同一批次产品应采集的样品件数；

c: 最大可允许超出 m 值的样品数；

m: 微生物指标可接受水平限量值（三级采样方案）或最高安全限量值（二级采样方案）；

M: 微生物指标的最高安全限量值；

金黄色葡萄球菌采用三级采样方案，其他微生物采用二级采样方案。

4.7　农药残留要求

应符合相关国家或地区对饮料类型产品中农药最大残留限量的规定。

5　试验方法

5.1　感官检验

应满足产品规格的要求。

5.2　理化检验

5.2.1　可溶性固形物

按 AOAC 932.14 或其他折光仪方法进行测试。

5.2.2　二氧化硫

按 AOAC 990.28 或其他蒸馏滴定方法进行测试。

5.3　污染物检验

5.3.1　砷、铅、汞、铜、锡

按 GB 5009.268 规定的方法测定，或其他国际通用 ICP/MS、AAS、ISO 方法进行测试，方法检出限满足符合性限值要求。

5.3.2　总黄曲霉毒素（B1、B2、G1、G2 之和）

按 GB 5009.22 或其他免疫亲和层析净化液相色谱法进行测试。

5.3.3　赭曲霉毒素 A

按 GB 5009.96 或其他免疫亲和层析净化液相色谱法进行测试。

5.4　微生物检验

5.4.1　菌落总数

按 ISO 4833–1 或其他 AOAC、ISO 等国际通用方法进行测试。

5.4.2　大肠菌群

按 ISO 4832 或其他 AOAC、ISO 等国际通用方法进行测试。

5.4.3　霉菌、酵母菌

按 FDA/BAM chapter 18 或其他 AOAC、ISO 等国际通用方法进行测试。

5.4.4　沙门氏菌

按 ISO 6579–1 或其他 AOAC、ISO 等国际通用方法进行测试。

5.4.5　金黄色葡萄球菌

按 AOAC 975.55 或其他 AOAC、ISO 等国际通用方法进行测试。

5.4.6　大肠杆菌

按 FDA/BAM chapter 4 或其他 AOAC、ISO 等国际通用方法进行测试。

5.4.7　商业无菌

按 GB 4789.26 或其他 AOAC、ISO 等国际通用方法进行测试。

6　标志

6.1　标签

应符合相关国家或地区预包装产品标签的规定。

营养成分及检测包括但不限于以下项目：能量、蛋白质、脂肪、（总）碳水化合物、钠、糖（单糖、双糖）或总糖、水分、灰分、反式脂肪、饱和脂肪、膳食纤维、维生素 D、胆固醇、钙、铁、钾、添加糖、糖醇等。

6.2　包装

应符合相关国家或地区的规定。

附录
（资料性附录）
凉茶饮料中最常用到的中药材原料

通用名称	基原（拉丁学名）	质量要求	参考来源
仙草	*Mesona chinensis* Benth.	符合相关国家或地区要求	《广东省中药志》
鸡蛋花	*Plumeria rubra* L. cv. Acutifolia	符合相关国家或地区要求	《广东省中药材标准第一册》
布渣叶	*Microcos paniculata* L.	符合相关国家或地区要求	《中国药典》
菊花	*Chrysanthemum morifolium* Ramat.	符合相关国家或地区要求	《中国药典》
金银花	*Lonicera japonica* Thunb.	符合相关国家或地区要求	《中国药典》《香港中药材标准》等
夏枯草	*Prunella vulgaris* L.	符合相关国家或地区要求	《中国药典》《香港中药材标准》等
甘草	*Glycyrrhiza uralensis* Fisch. *Glycyrrhiza inflata* Bat. *Glycyrrhiza glabra* L.	符合相关国家或地区要求	《中国药典》《美国药典》 《香港中药材标准》等
罗汉果	*Siraitia grosvenorii* (Swingle) C. Jeffrey ex A. M. Lu et Z. Y. Zhang	符合相关国家或地区要求	《中国药典》
桑叶	*Morus alba* L.	符合相关国家或地区要求	《中国药典》
淡竹叶	*Lophatherum gracile* Brongn.	符合相关国家或地区要求	《中国药典》
荷叶	*Nelumbo nucifera* Gaertn.	符合相关国家或地区要求	《中国药典》
青果	*Canarium album* Raeusch.	符合相关国家或地区要求	《中国药典》
槐花	*Sophora japonica* L.	符合相关国家或地区要求	《中国药典》
余甘子	*Phyllanthus emblica* L.	符合相关国家或地区要求	《中国药典》
茯苓	*Poria cocos* (Schw.) Wolf	符合相关国家或地区要求	《中国药典》
薏苡仁	*Coix lacryma-jobi* L. var. *mayuen* (Roman.) Stapf	符合相关国家或地区要求	《中国药典》
葛根	*Pueraria lobata* (Willd.) Ohwi	符合相关国家或地区要求	《中国药典》
桔梗	*Platycodon grandiflorum* (Jacq.) A. DC.	符合相关国家或地区要求	《中国药典》
马齿苋	*Portulaca oleracea* L.	符合相关国家或地区要求	《中国药典》
胖大海	*Sterculia lychnophora* Hance	符合相关国家或地区要求	《中国药典》
赤小豆	*Vigna umbellata* Ohwi et Ohashi *Vigna angularis* Ohwi et Ohashi	符合相关国家或地区要求	《中国药典》
莱菔子	*Raphanus sativus* L.	符合相关国家或地区要求	《中国药典》
玉竹	*Polygonatum odoratum* (Mill.) Druce	符合相关国家或地区要求	《中国药典》
山药	*Dioscorea opposita* Thunb.	符合相关国家或地区要求	《中国药典》

Foreword

Main Drafting Unit of this standard: SGS-CSTC Standards Technical Services Co., Ltd. Guangzhou Branch

Drafting Units participated: Guangzhou Wanglaoji Pharmaceutical Co., Ltd., Wanglaoji Great Health Industry Co., Ltd., Beijing Tongrentang (Bozhou) Prepared Slices of Chinese Crude Drugs CO., Ltd., Shenzhen Shenhui Enterprise Co., Ltd., Zhongshan Baiyi Drink Ltd., Puning Yi Junjia Food Co., Ltd., Guangxi Zhizhen Investment Co., Ltd., Nanyang Yuxing Beverage Co., Ltd., TRISTAR FOOD WHOLESALE CO INC. (USA), SHENG SHENG F&B INDUSTRIES PTE LTD. (Singapore)

Main Drafters of this standard: LI Chuyuan, ZHENG Rongbo, XU Wenliu, FANG Guanghong, YANG Lufang, HUANG Xiaodan, FENG Xiaoqing, QIU Yan, WENG Shaoquan, WU Bojian, PENG Shaozhong, LI Cizhou, ZHU Huanrong, SHEN Yingli, ZHANG Fengyuan, Ivan Chan (Hong Kong, China), Zhizheng REN (Taiwan, China), Michael G. Lien (USA), Charles Chua (Singapore)

Drafters and reviewers of this standard (in phonetic alphabetical order of last name):

China: Li Zhenji, Lin Ruichao, Chen Zhen, Han Jingyan, Fu Qiang, He Jieyi, Wei Jinming, Liu Xinlei, Chen Wenrui, Su Caizhu, Luo Jiani

Canada: Cheng Zhao

Spain: Chen Yueling, Ramon M. Calduch

Australia: Chijing Liu

Hungary: Gábor Nagy, Funian Yu, Linjun Xia

Ukraine: Samsonov

Iran: Amir Hooman Kazemi

Gabon: Ovonon Komo

Brazil: Reginaldo de Carvlaho Silva

Israel: Tuvia Scott

Italy: Hui Chen

New Zealand: Pengde Cui

USA: Deborah Lincoln, Haihe Tian

The drafting procedure of this standard complies with the SCM 0001-2009 *Working Regulations for Formulation and Publication of Standard* issued by the World Federation of Chinese Medicine Societies (WFCMS).

Liang Cha (Herbal Beverage)

1 Scope

This standard applies to pre-packaged Liang Cha (Herbal Beverage) as defined in 3.1.

2 Normative references

The following documents are referred to in the text in such a way that some or all of their content constitutes requirements of this document. For dated references, only the edition cited applies. For undated references, the latest edition of the referenced document (including any amendments) applies.

GB 4789.26 *National Standard for Food Safety —Microbiological Examination in Food: Commercial sterilization*

GB 5009.268 *National Standard for Food Safety —Determination of Multi-Elements in Food*

GB 5009.22 *National Standard for Food Safety —Determination of Aflatoxin Group B and G in Food*

GB 5009.96 *National Standard for Food Safety —Determination of Ochratoxin A in Food*

GB/T 22388 *Determination of melamine in raw milk and dairy products*

CAC/GL66 *Guidelines for the use of flavourings*

CODEX STAN *192 General standard for food additives*

CODEX STAN 193 *General standard for contaminants and toxins in food and feed*

AOAC 932.14 *Solids in syrups by means of refractometer*

AOAC 990.28 *Sulfites in foods optimized Monier-Williams method*

ISO 4833-1 *Microbiology of the food chain —Horizontal method for the enumeration of microorganisms —part 1: Colony count at 30℃ by the pour plate technique*

ISO 4832 *Microbiology of food and animal feeding stuffs —Horizontal method for the enumeration of coliforms —Colony-count technique*

ISO 6579-1 *Microbiology of the food chain —Horizontal method for the detection, enumeration and serotyping of Salmonella —Part 1: Detection of Salmonella spp*

FDA/BAM chapter 4 *Enumeration of Escherichia coli and the Coliform Bacteria*

AOAC 975.55 *Staphylococcus aureus in foods —surface plating method for isolation and enumeration*

ISO 18662-1 *Traditional Chinese medicine —Vocabulary —Part 1: Chinese Materia Medica.*

ISO 18664 *Traditional Chinese Medicine —Determination of heavy metals in herbal medicines used in Traditional Chinese Medicine*

ISO 21371 *Traditional Chinese medicine —Labeling requirements of products intended for oral or topical use*

FDA/BAM chapter 18 Yeasts, *Molds and Mycotoxins*

3 Term and definition

For the purposes of this standard, the following term and definition apply.

3.1 Liang Cha (Herbal Beverage)

Pre-packaged beverage based on the theory of the traditional Chinese Medicine, with one or more ingredients of grass jelly, frangipani, paniculate microcos leaf, chrysanthemum, etc. and other plant materials or extracts, and other ingredients or food additives are considered depending on the product, processed by extraction, concentration, preparation and sterilization, filling (or filling first before sterilization), packaging and other procedures.

4 Technical requirements

4.1 Raw and auxiliary and auxiliary materials requirements

Requirements for raw materials shall comply with corresponding standards, criteria and law and regulations in different countries and regions.

4.2 Sensory requirements

The product shall meet the sensory requirements such as specific color, smell and favor of the beverage prepared by the plants labeled.

4.3 Physical and chemical requirements

Physical and chemical requirements shall accord with the requirements in Table 1.

Table 1 Physical and chemical requirements

Items	Limits
Soluble solids	≥0.5g/L
SO_2 residue	≤10mg/L

4.4 Food additive requirements

Food additives shall comply with the food additives requirements of beverage in relevant countries and regions.

4.5 Contaminant requirements

Contaminants shall be in accordance with the requirements in Table 2.

Table 2 Contaminant requirements

Categories	Items	Limits
Heavy metals	Arsenic	≤0.1mg/ L
	Lead	≤0.2mg/ L
	Mercury	≤0.05mg/ L
	Copper	≤2.0mg/ L
	Tin (only applicable to canned products)	≤150mg/ L
Mycotoxins	Ochratoxin A	≤5μg/ L
	Total aflatoxins (sum of B1, B2, G1 and G2)	≤5μg/ L

4.6 Microbial indicator requirements

4.6.1 Microbial indicators of the caned products shall comply with the requirements of commercial sterilization.

4.6.2 Microbial indicators of other packaged products shall comply with the requirements in Table 3.

Table 3 Microbial Requirements

Items	Sampling scheme and quantity limit requirements			
	n	c	m	M
Total aerobic bacterial (CFU/mL)	5	0	200	/
Coliforms (CFU/mL)	5	0	0	/
Mold (CFU/mL)	≤20			
Yeast (CFU/mL)	≤20			
Salmonella (CFU /25mL)	5	0	0	/
Staphylococcal aureus (CFU/mL)	5	1	100	1000
Escherichia coli (CFU/mL)	5	0	0	/

Note:

n: the number of samples to be collected in one batch of products;

c: the maximum number of samples that can be allowed to exceed m value;

m: acceptable limited value for microbial indicators (the tertiary sampling scheme) or maximum safety limited value (the secondary sampling scheme);

M: maximum safety limited value of microbial indicators;

Three-stage sampling scheme is adopted for staphylococcal aureus, and the secondary sampling scheme is adopted for other microbes.

4.7 Pesticide residue requirements

Pesticide residue requirements shall be in accordance with standards and regulations of the maximum residue limits of pesticides for beverage products in corresponding countries and regions.

5 Test methods

5.1 Sensory test

Sensory test shall comply with the product specification requirements.

5.2 Physical and chemical test

5.2.1 Soluble solids

The test methods shall comply with the requirements given in AOAC 932.14 or other refractive methods.

5.2.2 Sulfur dioxide

The test methods shall comply with the requirements given in AOAC 990.28 or other distillation titration methods.

5.3 Contaminant test

5.3.1 Arsenic, Lead, Mercury, Copper and Tin

The test methods shall comply with the requirements in GB 5009.268 or other international general methods of ICP/MS or AAS or ISO. The detection limit of the method shall comply with the requirements of the compliance limit.

5.3.2 Total aflatoxins (sum of B1, B2, G1 and G2)

The test methods shall comply with the requirements in GB 5009.22 or other immunoaffinity chromatography purification liquid chromatography.

5.3.3 Ochratoxin A

The test methods shall comply with the requirements in GB 5009.96 or other immunoaffinity chromatography purification liquid chromatography.

5.4 Microbial test

5.4.1 Total aerobic bacterial count

The test methods shall comply with the requirements in ISO 4833-1 or other international general methods like AOAC and ISO.

5.4.2 Coliform count

The test methods shall comply with the requirements in ISO 4832 or other international general method like AOAC and ISO.

5.4.3 Mold, yeast

The test methods shall comply with the requirements in FDA/BAM chapter 18 or other international general methods like AOAC and ISO.

5.4.4 Salmonella

The test methods shall comply with the requirements in ISO 6579-1 or other international general method like AOAC and ISO.

5.4.5 Staphylococcal aureus (SA)

The test methods shall comply with the requirements in AOAC 975.55 or other international general methods like AOAC and ISO.

5.4.6 Escherichia coli

The test methods shall comply with the requirements in FDA/BAM chapter 4 or other international general methods like AOAC and ISO.

5.4.7 Commercial sterilization

The test methods shall comply with the requirements in GB 4789.26 or other international general method like AOAC and ISO.

6 Label and packaging

6.1 Label

The label of the products shall be in accordance with the regulations of pre-packaged product label in the relevant countries or regions.

Nutritional components and tests include but not limited to the following items: energy, protein, fat, (total) carbohydrate, sodium, sugar (monosaccharide, disaccharide) or total sugar, moisture, ash, trans fat, saturated fat, dietary fiber, Vitamin D, cholesterol, calcium, iron, potassium, added sugar, sugar alcohol, etc.

6.2 Packaging

The packaging of the products shall be in accordance with the regulations in relevant countries or regions.

Appendix
(Informative appendix)
The most commonly used raw Chinese medicinal in Liang Cha (Herbal Beverage)

Common Name	**Family & Genus (/Latin name)**	**Quality requirement**	**Reference source**
Grass Jelly	*Mesona chinensis* Benth.	Comply with the requirements of relevant countries or regions	*Journal of Chinese Materia Medica in Guangdong Province*
Frangipani	*Plumeria rubra* L. cv. Acutifolia	Comply with the requirements of relevant countries or regions	*Standard of Chinese Materia Medica in Guangdong Province* (Volume 1)
Paniculate Microcos Leaf	*Microcos paniculata L.*	Comply with the requirements of relevant countries or regions	*Pharmacopoeia of the People's Republic of China*
Chrysanthemum Flower	*Chrysanthemum morifolium* Ramat.	Comply with the requirements of relevant countries or regions	*Pharmacopoeia of the People's Republic of China*
Honeysuckle Flower	*Lonicera japonica* Thunb.	Comply with the requirements of relevant countries or regions	*Pharmacopoeia of the People's Republic of China, Hong Kong Standard for Chinese Materia Medica*, etc.
Common Selfheal Fruit-Spike	*Prunella vulgaris* L.	Comply with the requirements of relevant countries or regions	*Pharmacopoeia of the People's Republic of China, Hong Kong Standard for Chinese Materia medica*, etc.
Licorice Root	*Glycyrrhiza uralensis* Fisch. *Glycyrrhiza inflata* Bat. *Glycyrrhiza glabra* L.	Comply with the requirements of relevant countries or regions	*Pharmacopoeia of the People's Republic of China, American Herbal Pharmacopoeia, Hong Kong Standard for Chinese Materia Medica*, etc.
Grosvenor Momordica Fruit	*Siraitia grosvenorii* (Swingle) C. Jeffrey ex A. M. Lu et Z. Y. Zhang	Comply with the requirements of relevant countries or regions	*Pharmacopoeia of the People's Republic of China*
Mulberry Leaf	*Morus alba* L.	Comply with the requirements of relevant countries or regions	*Pharmacopoeia of the People's Republic of China*
Lophatherum Herb	*Lophatherum gracile* Brongn.	Comply with the requirements of relevant countries or regions	*Pharmacopoeia of the People's Republic of China*
Lotus Leaf	*Nelumbo nucifera* Gaertn.	Comply with the requirements of relevant countries or regions	*Pharmacopoeia of the People's Republic of China*

Common Name	Family & Genus (/Latin name)	Quality requirement	Reference source
Chinese White Olive	*Canarium album* Raeusch.	Comply with the requirements of relevant countries or regions	*Pharmacopoeia of the People's Republic of China*
Pagodatree Flower	*Sophora japonica* L.	Comply with the requirements of relevant countries or regions	*Pharmacopoeia of the People's Republic of China*
Emblic Leafflower Fruit	*Phyllanthus emblica* L.	Comply with the requirements of relevant countries or regions	*Pharmacopoeia of the People's Republic of China*
Indian Bread	*Poria cocos* (Schw.) Wolf	Comply with the requirements of relevant countries or regions	*Pharmacopoeia of the People's Republic of China*
Coix Seed	*Coix lacryma-jobi* L. var. *mayuen* (Roman.) Stapf	Comply with the requirements of relevant countries or regions	*Pharmacopoeia of the People's Republic of China*
Kudzuvine Root	*Pueraria lobata* (Willd.) Ohwi	Comply with the requirements of relevant countries or regions	*Pharmacopoeia of the People's Republic of China*
Platycodon Root	*Platycodon grandiflorum* (Jacq.) A. DC.	Comply with the requirements of relevant countries or regions	*Pharmacopoeia of the People's Republic of China*
Purslane Herb	*Portulaca oleracea* L.	Comply with the requirements of relevant countries or regions	*Pharmacopoeia of the People's Republic of China*
Boat-Fruited Sterculia Seed	*Sterculia lychnophora* Hance	Comply with the requirements of relevant countries or regions	*Pharmacopoeia of the People's Republic of China*
Rice Bean	*Vigna umbellata* Ohwi et Ohashi *Vigna angularis* Ohwi et Ohashi	Comply with the requirements of relevant countries or regions	*Pharmacopoeia of the People's Republic of China*
Radish Seed	*Raphanus sativus* L.	Comply with the requirements of relevant countries or regions	*Pharmacopoeia of the People's Republic of China*
Fragrant Solomonseal Rhizome	*Polygonatum odoratum* (Mill.) Druce	Comply with the requirements of relevant countries or regions	*Pharmacopoeia of the People's Republic of China*
Common Yam Rhizome	*Dioscorea opposita* Thunb.	Comply with the requirements of relevant countries or regions	*Pharmacopoeia of the People's Republic of China*